If Lost, Please Contact:

Name:_____

Phone:_____

A Goal
Without A Plan
Is Just
A Wish

DEDICATION

This ENTER THE FASTING LANE Intermittent Fasting Journal is dedicated to all the new and dedicated fasters out there who are full of excitement & passion from seeing daily, weekly & monthly progress towards their goals! We know that daily fasting takes work and time and is HARD, but the journey is worth it! We are honored to be a part of that in any small way!

YOU are my inspiration for producing these fasting books and I'm honored to be a part of keeping all of your fasting experiences and notes organized all in one easy to find spot!

HOW TO USE

This Enter The Fasting Lane Journal is the perfect daily fasting tracker!

1. Reflect on why you are fasting.
2. Write your thoughts and feelings daily.
3. Write or underline any lessons learned. Summarize any lessons learned for easier memory.
4. If you start obsessing over food, try brushing your teeth or walking.
5. Set daily, monthly & weekly goals.
6. Share your findings with others and become a resource!

Day 1

IN THE BEGINNING	
Date	
Weight	
Chest	
Arm	
Waist	
Hips	

Weekly Goals

Daily Fasting Hours:_____

Daily Water Intake:_____

Daily Calories:_____

Daily Carbs:_____

Daily Exercise:

My Motivation For The Week

_____
_____
_____
_____
_____
_____
_____
_____
_____
_____
_____

Day 1
Date:

START FAST	END FAST	TOTAL FAST TIME
AM/PM	AM/PM	

Fast Broken With:

_____

Meal 1

Food/Beverage	Cals	Carbs	Fat	Protein
SUBTOTALS				

Meal 2

Food/Beverage	Cals	Carbs	Fat	Protein
SUBTOTALS				

Water Intake

Daily Notes

_____
_____
_____
_____
_____
_____
_____
_____
_____
_____
_____
_____
_____
_____
_____
_____
_____
_____
_____
_____
_____
_____
_____

Day 2
Date:

START FAST AM/PM	END FAST AM/PM	TOTAL FAST TIME

Fast Broken With:
_____

Meal 1

Food/Beverage	Cals	Carbs	Fat	Protein
SUBTOTALS				

Meal 2

Food/Beverage	Cals	Carbs	Fat	Protein
SUBTOTALS				

Water Intake

Daily Notes

_____
_____
_____
_____
_____
_____
_____
_____
_____
_____
_____
_____
_____
_____
_____
_____
_____
_____
_____
_____
_____
_____
_____
_____

Day 3
Date:

START FAST AM/PM	END FAST AM/PM	TOTAL FAST TIME

Fast Broken With:
_____

Meal 1

Food/Beverage	Cals	Carbs	Fat	Protein
SUBTOTALS				

Meal 2

Food/Beverage	Cals	Carbs	Fat	Protein
SUBTOTALS				

Water Intake

Daily Notes

_____
_____
_____
_____
_____
_____
_____
_____
_____
_____
_____
_____
_____
_____
_____
_____
_____
_____
_____
_____
_____

Day 4
Date:

START FAST AM/PM	END FAST AM/PM	TOTAL FAST TIME

Fast Broken With:
_____

Meal 1

Food/Beverage	Cals	Carbs	Fat	Protein
SUBTOTALS				

Meal 2

Food/Beverage	Cals	Carbs	Fat	Protein
SUBTOTALS				

Water Intake

Daily Notes

Day 5
Date:

START FAST AM/PM	END FAST AM/PM	TOTAL FAST TIME

Fast Broken With:
_____

Meal 1

Food/Beverage	Cals	Carbs	Fat	Protein
SUBTOTALS				

Meal 2

Food/Beverage	Cals	Carbs	Fat	Protein
SUBTOTALS				

Water Intake

Daily Notes

Day 6
Date:

START FAST	END FAST	TOTAL FAST TIME
AM/PM	AM/PM	

Fast Broken With:
_____

Meal 1

Food/Beverage	Cals	Carbs	Fat	Protein
SUBTOTALS				

Meal 2

Food/Beverage	Cals	Carbs	Fat	Protein
SUBTOTALS				

Water Intake

Daily Notes

Day 7
Date:

START FAST AM/PM	END FAST AM/PM	TOTAL FAST TIME

Fast Broken With:
_____

Meal 1

Food/Beverage	Cals	Carbs	Fat	Protein
SUBTOTALS				

Meal 2

Food/Beverage	Cals	Carbs	Fat	Protein
SUBTOTALS				

Weekly Recap

Week 1 Success

Date	
Weight	
Chest	
Arm	
Waist	
Hips	

Daily Fasting Hours Achieved?_____

Daily Water Intake Achieved?_____

Daily Calories Achieved?_____

Daily Carbs Achieved?_____

Daily Exercise Achieved?_____

Struggles This Week

_____
_____
_____
_____

Successes This Week

_____
_____
_____
_____

Notes

_____
_____
_____
_____
_____
_____
_____
_____
_____
_____
_____
_____
_____
_____
_____
_____
_____
_____
_____
_____

Weekly Goals

Daily Fasting Hours:_____

Daily Water Intake:_____

Daily Calories:_____

Daily Carbs:_____

Daily Exercise:

My Motivation For The Week

_____
_____
_____
_____
_____
_____
_____
_____
_____
_____
_____
_____

Day 8
Date:

START FAST	END FAST	TOTAL FAST TIME
AM/PM	AM/PM	

Fast Broken With:
_____

Meal 1

Food/Beverage	Cals	Carbs	Fat	Protein
SUBTOTALS				

Meal 2

Food/Beverage	Cals	Carbs	Fat	Protein
SUBTOTALS				

Water Intake

Daily Notes

Day 9
Date:

START FAST AM/PM	END FAST AM/PM	TOTAL FAST TIME

Fast Broken With:
_____

Meal 1

Food/Beverage	Cals	Carbs	Fat	Protein
SUBTOTALS				

Meal 2

Food/Beverage	Cals	Carbs	Fat	Protein
SUBTOTALS				

Water Intake

Daily Notes

Day 10
Date:

START FAST	END FAST	TOTAL FAST TIME
AM/PM	AM/PM	

Fast Broken With:
_____

Meal 1

Food/Beverage	Cals	Carbs	Fat	Protein
SUBTOTALS				

Meal 2

Food/Beverage	Cals	Carbs	Fat	Protein
SUBTOTALS				

Water Intake

Daily Notes

_____
_____
_____
_____
_____
_____
_____
_____
_____
_____
_____
_____
_____
_____
_____
_____
_____
_____
_____
_____
_____
_____

Day 11
Date:

START FAST AM/PM	END FAST AM/PM	TOTAL FAST TIME

Fast Broken With:
_____

Meal 1

Food/Beverage	Cals	Carbs	Fat	Protein
SUBTOTALS				

Meal 2

Food/Beverage	Cals	Carbs	Fat	Protein
SUBTOTALS				

Water Intake

☐ ☐ ☐ ☐ ☐ ☐ ☐ ☐ ☐

Daily Notes

_____
_____
_____
_____
_____
_____
_____
_____
_____
_____
_____
_____
_____
_____
_____
_____
_____
_____
_____
_____
_____
_____
_____

Day 12
Date:

START FAST AM/PM	END FAST AM/PM	TOTAL FAST TIME

Fast Broken With:
_____

Meal 1

Food/Beverage	Cals	Carbs	Fat	Protein
SUBTOTALS				

Meal 2

Food/Beverage	Cals	Carbs	Fat	Protein
SUBTOTALS				

Water Intake

Daily Notes

Day 13
Date:

START FAST AM/PM	END FAST AM/PM	TOTAL FAST TIME

Fast Broken With:
_____

Meal 1

Food/Beverage	Cals	Carbs	Fat	Protein
SUBTOTALS				

Meal 2

Food/Beverage	Cals	Carbs	Fat	Protein
SUBTOTALS				

Water Intake

Daily Notes

_____
_____
_____
_____
_____
_____
_____
_____
_____
_____
_____
_____
_____
_____
_____
_____
_____
_____
_____
_____
_____
_____
_____
_____

Day 14
Date:

START FAST AM/PM	END FAST AM/PM	TOTAL FAST TIME

Fast Broken With:
_____

Meal 1

Food/Beverage	Cals	Carbs	Fat	Protein
SUBTOTALS				

Meal 2

Food/Beverage	Cals	Carbs	Fat	Protein
SUBTOTALS				

Water Intake

Daily Notes

Weekly Recap

Week 2 Success

Date	
Weight	
Chest	
Arm	
Waist	
Hips	

Daily Fasting Hours Achieved?_____

Daily Water Intake Achieved?_____

Daily Calories Achieved?_____

Daily Carbs Achieved?_____

Daily Exercise Achieved?_____

Struggles This Week

_____
_____
_____
_____

Successes This Week

Notes

Weekly Goals

Daily Fasting Hours: _____

Daily Water Intake: _____

Daily Calories: _____

Daily Carbs: _____

Daily Exercise: _____

My Motivation For The Week

_____
_____
_____
_____
_____
_____
_____
_____
_____
_____
_____
_____

Day 15
Date:

START FAST AM/PM	END FAST AM/PM	TOTAL FAST TIME

Fast Broken With:
_____

Meal 1

Food/Beverage	Cals	Carbs	Fat	Protein
SUBTOTALS				

Meal 2

Food/Beverage	Cals	Carbs	Fat	Protein
SUBTOTALS				

Water Intake

Daily Notes

_____
_____
_____
_____
_____
_____
_____
_____
_____
_____
_____
_____
_____
_____
_____
_____
_____
_____
_____
_____
_____
_____

Day 16
Date:

START FAST AM/PM	END FAST AM/PM	TOTAL FAST TIME

Fast Broken With:
_____

Meal 1

Food/Beverage	Cals	Carbs	Fat	Protein
SUBTOTALS				

Meal 2

Food/Beverage	Cals	Carbs	Fat	Protein
SUBTOTALS				

Water Intake

Daily Notes

Day 17
Date:

START FAST AM/PM	END FAST AM/PM	TOTAL FAST TIME

Fast Broken With:
_____

Meal 1

Food/Beverage	Cals	Carbs	Fat	Protein
SUBTOTALS				

Meal 2

Food/Beverage	Cals	Carbs	Fat	Protein
SUBTOTALS				

Water Intake

Daily Notes

_____
_____
_____
_____
_____
_____
_____
_____
_____
_____
_____
_____
_____
_____
_____
_____
_____
_____
_____
_____
_____
_____

Day 18
Date:

START FAST AM/PM	END FAST AM/PM	TOTAL FAST TIME

Fast Broken With:
_____

Meal 1

Food/Beverage	Cals	Carbs	Fat	Protein
SUBTOTALS				

Meal 2

Food/Beverage	Cals	Carbs	Fat	Protein
SUBTOTALS				

Water Intake

Daily Notes

Day 19
Date:

START FAST AM/PM	END FAST AM/PM	TOTAL FAST TIME

Fast Broken With:
_____

Meal 1

Food/Beverage	Cals	Carbs	Fat	Protein
SUBTOTALS				

Meal 2

Food/Beverage	Cals	Carbs	Fat	Protein
SUBTOTALS				

Water Intake

Daily Notes

_____
_____
_____
_____
_____
_____
_____
_____
_____
_____
_____
_____
_____
_____
_____
_____
_____
_____
_____
_____
_____
_____
_____
_____
_____

Day 20
Date:

START FAST	END FAST	TOTAL FAST TIME
AM/PM	AM/PM	

Fast Broken With:

_____

Meal 1

Food/Beverage	Cals	Carbs	Fat	Protein
SUBTOTALS				

Meal 2

Food/Beverage	Cals	Carbs	Fat	Protein
SUBTOTALS				

Water Intake

Daily Notes

Day 21
Date:

START FAST AM/PM	END FAST AM/PM	TOTAL FAST TIME

Fast Broken With:
_____

Meal 1

Food/Beverage	Cals	Carbs	Fat	Protein
SUBTOTALS				

Meal 2

Food/Beverage	Cals	Carbs	Fat	Protein
SUBTOTALS				

Water Intake

Daily Notes

Weekly Recap

Week 3 Success

Date	
Weight	
Chest	
Arm	
Waist	
Hips	

Daily Fasting Hours Achieved?_____

Daily Water Intake Achieved?_____

Daily Calories Achieved?_____

Daily Carbs Achieved?_____

Daily Exercise Achieved?_____

Struggles This Week

_____

_____

_____

_____

Successes This Week

Notes

Weekly Goals

Daily Fasting Hours:_____

Daily Water Intake:_____

Daily Calories:_____

Daily Carbs:_____

Daily Exercise:

My Motivation For The Week

_____
_____
_____
_____
_____
_____
_____
_____
_____
_____
_____

Date: Day 22

START FAST AM/PM	END FAST AM/PM	TOTAL FAST TIME

Fast Broken With:

_____

Meal 1

Food/Beverage	Cals	Carbs	Fat	Protein
SUBTOTALS				

Meal 2

Food/Beverage	Cals	Carbs	Fat	Protein
SUBTOTALS				

Water Intake

Daily Notes

_____
_____
_____
_____
_____
_____
_____
_____
_____
_____
_____
_____
_____
_____
_____
_____
_____
_____
_____
_____
_____
_____

Day 23
Date:

START FAST AM/PM	END FAST AM/PM	TOTAL FAST TIME

Fast Broken With:
_____

Meal 1

Food/Beverage	Cals	Carbs	Fat	Protein
SUBTOTALS				

Meal 2

Food/Beverage	Cals	Carbs	Fat	Protein
SUBTOTALS				

Water Intake

Daily Notes

_____
_____
_____
_____
_____
_____
_____
_____
_____
_____
_____
_____
_____
_____
_____
_____
_____
_____
_____
_____
_____
_____
_____

Day 24
Date:

START FAST AM/PM	END FAST AM/PM	TOTAL FAST TIME

Fast Broken With:
_____

Meal 1

Food/Beverage	Cals	Carbs	Fat	Protein
SUBTOTALS				

Meal 2

Food/Beverage	Cals	Carbs	Fat	Protein
SUBTOTALS				

Water Intake

Daily Notes

Day 25
Date:

START FAST AM/PM	END FAST AM/PM	TOTAL FAST TIME

Fast Broken With:
_____

Meal 1

Food/Beverage	Cals	Carbs	Fat	Protein
SUBTOTALS				

Meal 2

Food/Beverage	Cals	Carbs	Fat	Protein
SUBTOTALS				

Water Intake

☐ ☐ ☐ ☐ ☐ ☐ ☐ ☐

Daily Notes

_____
_____
_____
_____
_____
_____
_____
_____
_____
_____
_____
_____
_____
_____
_____
_____
_____
_____
_____
_____
_____
_____

Day 26
Date:

START FAST AM/PM	END FAST AM/PM	TOTAL FAST TIME

Fast Broken With:
_____

Meal 1

Food/Beverage	Cals	Carbs	Fat	Protein
SUBTOTALS				

Meal 2

Food/Beverage	Cals	Carbs	Fat	Protein
SUBTOTALS				

Water Intake

Daily Notes

_____
_____
_____
_____
_____
_____
_____
_____
_____
_____
_____
_____
_____
_____
_____
_____
_____
_____
_____
_____

Day 27
Date:

START FAST	END FAST	TOTAL FAST TIME
AM/PM	AM/PM	

Fast Broken With:
_____

Meal 1

Food/Beverage	Cals	Carbs	Fat	Protein
SUBTOTALS				

Meal 2

Food/Beverage	Cals	Carbs	Fat	Protein
SUBTOTALS				

Water Intake

Daily Notes

_____
_____
_____
_____
_____
_____
_____
_____
_____
_____
_____
_____
_____
_____
_____
_____
_____
_____
_____
_____
_____
_____
_____
_____

Day 28
Date:

START FAST	END FAST	TOTAL FAST TIME
AM/PM	AM/PM	

Fast Broken With:
_____

Meal 1

Food/Beverage	Cals	Carbs	Fat	Protein
SUBTOTALS				

Meal 2

Food/Beverage	Cals	Carbs	Fat	Protein
SUBTOTALS				

Water Intake

Daily Notes

_____
_____
_____
_____
_____
_____
_____
_____
_____
_____
_____
_____
_____
_____
_____
_____
_____
_____
_____
_____
_____
_____
_____
_____
_____

Weekly Recap

Week 3 Success

Date

Weight

Chest

Arm

Waist

Hips

Daily Fasting Hours Achieved?_____

Daily Water Intake Achieved?_____

Daily Calories Achieved?_____

Daily Carbs Achieved?_____

Daily Exercise Achieved?_____

Struggles This Week

_____

_____

_____

_____

Successes This Week

Notes

Weekly Goals

Daily Fasting Hours:_____

Daily Water Intake:_____

Daily Calories:_____

Daily Carbs:_____

Daily Exercise:

My Motivation For The Week

_____
_____
_____
_____
_____
_____
_____
_____
_____
_____
_____
_____
_____

Day 29
Date:

START FAST AM/PM	END FAST AM/PM	TOTAL FAST TIME

Fast Broken With:

_____

Meal 1

Food/Beverage	Cals	Carbs	Fat	Protein
SUBTOTALS				

Meal 2

Food/Beverage	Cals	Carbs	Fat	Protein
SUBTOTALS				

Water Intake

Daily Notes

_____
_____
_____
_____
_____
_____
_____
_____
_____
_____
_____
_____
_____
_____
_____
_____
_____
_____
_____
_____
_____
_____

Day 30
Date:

START FAST AM/PM	END FAST AM/PM	TOTAL FAST TIME

Fast Broken With:
_____

Meal 1

Food/Beverage	Cals	Carbs	Fat	Protein
SUBTOTALS				

Meal 2

Food/Beverage	Cals	Carbs	Fat	Protein
SUBTOTALS				

Water Intake

Daily Notes

Day 31
Date:

START FAST AM/PM	END FAST AM/PM	TOTAL FAST TIME

Fast Broken With:
_____

Meal 1

Food/Beverage	Cals	Carbs	Fat	Protein
SUBTOTALS				

Meal 2

Food/Beverage	Cals	Carbs	Fat	Protein
SUBTOTALS				

Water Intake

Daily Notes

Monthly Recap

Monthly Success

Date	
Weight	
Chest	
Arm	
Waist	
Hips	

Daily Fasting Hours Achieved?_____

Daily Water Intake Achieved?_____

Daily Calories Achieved?_____

Daily Carbs Achieved?_____

Daily Exercise Achieved?_____

Struggles This Month

_____
_____
_____
_____

Successes This Month

_____
_____
_____

_____

Notes

_____
_____
_____
_____
_____
_____
_____
_____
_____
_____
_____
_____
_____
_____
_____
_____
_____
_____
_____
_____
_____

Day 30

A BEAUTIFUL ENDING

Date	
Weight	
Chest	
Arm	
Waist	
Hips	

Journal

Journal

Journal

Journal

Journal

Journal

Journal

Journal

Journal

Journal

www.ingramcontent.com/pod-product-compliance
Lightning Source LLC
Chambersburg PA
CBHW071724020426
42333CB00017B/2387